THE MUMPS VIRUS AND TREATMENT

Understanding The Cause of The Infectious Disease Recognizing Their Symptoms And Knowing How To Prevent From Spreading.

Becky Rowland

Copyright © 2024 by [Becky Rowland]

All rights reserved. No part of this publication may be reproduced, distributed, or transmitted in any form or by any means, including photocopying, recording, or other electronic or mechanical methods, without the prior written permission of the publisher, except in the case of brief quotations embodied in critical reviews and certain other noncommercial uses permitted by copyright law.

I

Introduction

    Definition of Mumps

    Importance Of Understanding The Virus And Its Treatment

II

The Mumps Virus

    Description of the Mumps Virus

    How The Virus Spreads

    Symptoms Of Mumps

III

Diagnosis Of Mumps

    Physical Examination And Medical History

    Recommended Tests

IV

Treatment Options for Mumps

    General Approach(Since Mumps Usually Resolves On Its Own)

    Medications For Symptom Relief

    Lifestyle Changes And Home Remedies For Mumps

V

Complications Of Mumps

    Rare But Serious Complications - Orchitis, Pancreatitis, Oophoritis, Mastitis Encephalitis, Meningitis

VI

Prevention Of Mumps

    Mumps Vaccination

    Characteristics

    Vaccination Schedule And Use

- Vaccination Of Adults
- Revaccination
- Vaccination During Mumps Outbreaks
- Mumps Immunity
- Immunogenicity And Vaccine Efficacy

VII

Conclusion
- Summary of Key Points
- The Significance Of Vaccination And Early Treatment

I

Introduction

Definition of Mumps

Mumps is a contagious viral infection primarily known for causing painful swellings at the side of the face under the ears (the parotid glands), leading to a distinctive "hamster-like" appearance. This illness, which has affected populations globally, is caused by the mumps virus, a member of the paramyxovirus family. It spreads through direct contact with respiratory secretions or saliva from an infected person.

In the fifth century BCE, Hippocrates wrote a description of parotitis and orchitis. A filterable substance found in saliva was the cause of mumps, as Claud Johnson and Ernest Goodpasture proved in 1934 when they showed that the disease could be spread from sick humans to rhesus monkeys. In 1935, the viral nature of this agent was revealed. Prior to the development of a vaccine in 1967, mumps was one of the most frequent causes of aseptic meningitis and sensorineural hearing loss in children in the United States.

Understanding mumps goes beyond its medical definition; it's about recognizing a health adversary that has been both a childhood rite of passage and a public health challenge. The virus's ability to spread quickly through communities, especially among those who are unvaccinated, underscores the importance of awareness and prevention. The characteristic symptoms of mumps, such as fever, headache, muscle aches, fatigue, and loss of appetite, typically appear two to three weeks after exposure to the virus and are often followed by the swelling of the parotid glands.

Importance Of Understanding The Virus And Its Treatment

Grasping the significance of understanding mumps is crucial for several reasons. Firstly, while mumps is often mild, it can lead to serious complications, such as inflammation of the brain (encephalitis) and reproductive organs, which can have long-term consequences. Secondly, the knowledge of mumps and its treatment options empowers individuals to seek timely medical care, thereby reducing the risk of complications.

Treatment for mumps is primarily supportive, as the body usually clears the virus on its own. However, knowing how to alleviate symptoms and prevent transmission during the infectious period can significantly impact individual comfort and community health. This includes using analgesics for pain and fever, applying warm or cold compresses to reduce gland swelling, and ensuring adequate hydration and rest.

Moreover, understanding mumps extends to recognizing the role of vaccination in disease prevention. The measles-mumps-rubella (MMR) vaccine has dramatically reduced the incidence of mumps, making it a rare occurrence in many parts of the world. However, outbreaks can still happen, particularly in settings where individuals are in close contact, such as schools and colleges. Therefore, maintaining high vaccination rates is essential to prevent the spread of mumps and protect those who are most vulnerable.

In summary, the definition of mumps and the importance of understanding the virus and its treatment are intertwined in the broader context of public health. It's a narrative that emphasizes the power of knowledge, the importance of prevention, and the value of compassionate care in the face of illness.

II

The Mumps Virus

Description of the Mumps Virus

The mumps virus, a stealthy infiltrator of our daily lives, is an entity that has long been a part of human history. It's a member of the paramyxovirus family, a group of viruses that are known for their ability to spread rapidly and cause a range of respiratory illnesses. The mumps virus is particularly adept at targeting our salivary glands, especially the parotid glands, leading to the characteristic swelling that has become synonymous with the disease.

This virus is not just a cluster of RNA and proteins; it's a challenge to our collective health and a reminder of our vulnerability. Its structure is simple yet effective, allowing it to bind to our cells and replicate within them. The mumps virus contains a single-stranded RNA genome, which it uses to hijack the host cell's machinery to produce more copies of itself. The virus's outer shell, or envelope, helps it to enter and exit our cells, continuing its cycle of infection and spread.

Understanding the mumps virus is akin to learning the tactics of an opponent. It's about knowing its strengths and weaknesses, its methods of attack, and how it can be stopped. This knowledge is not just academic; it's a crucial part of our defense against a virus that has the potential to disrupt lives and communities.

How The Virus Spreads

The mumps virus is a master of movement, finding its way from one person to another with ease. It travels in the droplets expelled when an infected person coughs or sneezes, turning the air we breathe into a pathway for diseases. These droplets can land on surfaces, where the virus lies in wait to be picked up by the next unsuspecting individual.

But the virus's reach extends beyond the air. It thrives in the saliva of an infected person, making sharing utensils or drinks a common route for its journey. Even the simple act of touching a contaminated surface and then touching one's face can be enough to invite the virus in. Person-to-person contact is the virus's preferred mode of travel. A handshake, a hug, or a kiss can all be conduits for the mumps virus, as it seeks out new hosts to infect. It's a reminder of the intimacy of human interaction and the care we must take to protect ourselves and others.

The spread of the mumps virus is not just a matter of biology; it's a narrative of our interconnectedness. It shows us how our actions have consequences, not just for ourselves, but for the health of our communities. By understanding how the virus spreads, we arm ourselves with the knowledge to break the chain of transmission and keep our communities safe.

In conclusion, the mumps virus is a formidable adversary, but it is one that we can understand and combat. Through vigilance, vaccination, and education, we can ensure that the story of the mumps virus is one of triumph, not tragedy.

Symptoms Of Mumps

Mumps, a viral illness that once was a common childhood ailment, has become less prevalent due to the advent of vaccinations. Yet, when it does appear, it brings with it a suite of symptoms that are unmistakable and often uncomfortable.

- **Swelling Of Parotid Glands**

The most recognizable sign of mumps is the swelling of the parotid glands, which are the largest of the salivary glands. Located just below and in front of the ears, these glands can swell to the point where they push the lobes of the ears outward and up. This swelling can cause discomfort and pain, particularly when chewing or swallowing.

The inflammation of these glands, known as parotitis, can be unilateral or bilateral. When bilateral, it gives the face a rounded, puffed appearance that is often referred to colloquially as "chipmunk cheeks." The skin over the swollen glands may appear stretched and shiny, and the area can be warm to the touch. This swelling typically develops within the first two days of infection and can last for a week or more.

- **Fever, Headache, Muscle Ache**

Accompanying the swelling of the glands are systemic symptoms that can mimic those of the flu. Fever is often the first to present, sometimes reaching as high as 103°F (39°C). It serves as the body's natural defense mechanism, attempting to create an environment less hospitable to the virus.

Headaches, ranging from dull to severe, can be persistent and debilitating. They are often exacerbated by the pressure from the swollen glands. Muscle aches, particularly in the proximal muscles like those of the back and neck, can add to the overall feeling of malaise. These aches are the body's response to the viral invasion, signaling an immune response.

- **Loss Of Appetite, Weakness, And Fatigue**

As the body diverts energy to fight off the mumps virus, patients often experience a loss of appetite. This can be due to a combination of factors, including the pain from swollen glands, general discomfort from fever, and the body's focus on immune response rather than digestion.

Weakness and fatigue are also common, as the body's resources are consumed by the effort to combat the virus. Patients may feel exhausted and find it difficult to perform even simple tasks. Rest becomes a crucial component of recovery, as the body needs to conserve energy for the immune battle.

In conclusion, the symptoms of mumps, while uncomfortable, are a testament to the body's resilience and ability to fight off viral invaders. Understanding these symptoms can help in recognizing the illness early and taking steps to manage the discomfort and prevent the spread of the virus.

III

Diagnosis Of Mumps

Physical Examination And Medical History

When a patient presents with symptoms suggestive of mumps, the first step in the diagnostic journey is a thorough physical examination and review of medical history. The healthcare provider looks for the classic signs of mumps, such as the swelling of the parotid glands, while also inquiring about recent health events that might point to mumps exposure.

The medical history is a tapestry of the patient's health, woven with threads of past illnesses, vaccinations, and exposures. It provides context to the present condition, offering clues that guide the healthcare provider towards a diagnosis. A history of exposure to someone with mumps or a lack of vaccination against the virus can be particularly telling.

Recommended Tests

Once the initial examination and history suggest mumps, specific tests are recommended to confirm the diagnosis. These tests are designed to detect the presence of the mumps virus or the body's response to it.

- **Antibody Test**

The antibody test is a key player in the diagnostic process. It detects antibodies, which are proteins produced by the immune system in response to the mumps virus. There are two types of antibodies that the test looks for: IgM and IgG. IgM antibodies indicate a recent infection, while IgG antibodies suggest past exposure or vaccination.

The timing of the test is crucial, as the presence of IgM antibodies is highest shortly after the onset of symptoms. However, in individuals who have been vaccinated, the detection of IgM can be more challenging, and a negative result does not necessarily rule out mumps.

- **Culture Test**

The culture test takes a different approach. It involves growing the virus from a sample taken from the patient, usually from the mouth or throat. This test can provide definitive evidence of the virus, but it requires time—often several weeks—for the virus to grow enough to be detected.

The culture test is less commonly used due to the time it takes and the availability of more rapid tests. However, in certain cases, such as when other tests are inconclusive or when a more detailed analysis of the virus is needed, a culture can be invaluable.

In conclusion, the diagnosis of mumps is a multifaceted process that combines clinical assessment with targeted testing.

Each step, from the initial examination to the recommended tests, builds upon the last, culminating in a comprehensive understanding of the patient's condition. It's a process that exemplifies the blend of art and science that is medicine, all aimed at providing the best care for the patient.

IV

Treatment Options for Mumps

General Approach (Since Mumps Usually Resolves On Its Own)

Mumps, a viral encounter that often takes us by surprise, is typically a self-limiting illness. This means that in most cases, the body's immune system will clear the virus without the need for medical intervention. The general approach to managing mumps centers on providing comfort during the course of the illness and minimizing the risk of spreading the virus to others.

Rest is paramount. The body needs energy to fight off the infection, and rest provides the necessary respite for the immune system to do its work effectively. Patients are encouraged to stay home, avoid strenuous activities, and get plenty of sleep.

Hydration is another cornerstone of the general approach. Fever and salivary gland swelling can lead to dehydration, so it's important to drink ample fluids. Water, fruit juices, and broths are excellent choices to maintain hydration levels.

Isolation is recommended to prevent the spread of the virus. Since mumps is contagious, patients should avoid close contact with others, especially during the first five days after the onset of gland swelling.

Medications For Symptom Relief

While there is no cure for mumps, medications can be used to alleviate the symptoms. Over-the-counter pain relievers like acetaminophen and ibuprofen are effective in reducing fever and relieving pain. These medications can help manage the discomfort from swollen glands, headaches, and general body aches.

Acetaminophen is known for its fever-reducing and pain-relieving properties. It's a suitable option for those who need to manage fever and pain without the anti-inflammatory effects.

Ibuprofen, on the other hand, not only reduces fever and relieves pain but also offers anti-inflammatory benefits. This can be particularly helpful in reducing the inflammation associated with swollen glands.

It's important to use these medications as directed and to consult with a healthcare provider before starting any new medication, especially if the patient has other health conditions or is taking other medications.

In conclusion, the treatment for mumps is largely supportive, focusing on rest, hydration, isolation, and symptom relief. By following these guidelines, patients can ensure a more comfortable recovery period and help prevent the spread of the virus to others. Remember, while mumps is usually a mild illness, it's always wise to consult with a healthcare provider for personalized advice and care.

Lifestyle Changes And Home Remedies For Mumps

Rest And Isolation

When mumps enter a household, it demands a pause in the rhythm of daily life. Rest becomes not just a recommendation, but a necessity. The body, engaged in an invisible battle against the virus, requires downtime to marshal its defenses and repair the collateral damage of the immune response. Patients are advised to retreat from the bustle of their routines, to find solace in the quiet corners of their homes, where healing can begin.

Isolation, too, is a critical component of the recovery process—not just for the one who is ill, but for the community at large. Mumps, a contagion that thrives on proximity, is halted by distance. Those affected are counseled to keep to themselves, to become temporary islands in the stream of social interaction. This separation is a gesture of responsibility, a silent acknowledgment of the interconnectedness of health.

Warm Or Cold Compresses

The debate between warmth and cold is as old as remedies themselves. For the swollen visage of mumps, both have their place. Warm compresses, gentle and soothing, can ease the discomfort of swollen glands, like a soft whisper against the skin, telling the inflamed tissues to relax. Cold compresses, on the other hand, bring the sharp clarity of ice, numbing the pain and reducing inflammation, a stern command for swelling to recede.

The choice between the two is personal, a conversation between the patient and their own body. Some find relief in the embrace of warmth; others, in the brisk shock of cold. Both are allies in the journey to wellness, simple yet profound tools in the human arsenal against discomfort.

Soft Foods And Plenty Of Fluids

Nutrition during the time of mumps is a delicate dance. The act of chewing, typically thoughtless, becomes a calculated maneuver, navigating the tender landscape of a swollen mouth. Soft foods—creamy potatoes, runny oatmeal, rice porridge—become staples, their textures forgiving, requiring minimal effort from the weary jaws.

Fluids, too, take on new importance. They are the carriers of life, the medium through which nutrients flow, and waste departs. In the fevered state of illness, they replenish what the body loses in heat, ensuring that the machinery of life does not grind to a halt from lack of hydration.

In this chapter of illness, the kitchen becomes an apothecary, the spoon, a vessel of healing. Each meal is a step on the path to recovery, each sip, a small victory in the fight against the virus.

In conclusion, the journey through mumps is one of retreat, comfort, and nourishment. It is a time when the body asks for patience, and the world obliges, slowing its pace to the rhythm of healing.

V

Complications Of Mumps

Rare But Serious Complications - Orchitis, Pancreatitis, Oophoritis, Mastitis Encephalitis, Meningitis

Orchitis

Orchitis is an inflammation of the testicles that can occur as a complication of mumps, particularly in post-pubertal males. It typically develops 4 to 8 days after the onset of mumps symptoms and can result in severe pain, swelling, and, in some cases, reduced fertility. While most individuals recover without long-term effects, some may experience atrophy of the testicles or decreased sperm production.

Pancreatitis

Pancreatitis due to mumps is characterized by inflammation of the pancreas, leading to abdominal pain, nausea, and vomiting. This condition is generally temporary and resolves as the mumps infection subsides. However, in severe cases, it may require hospitalization to support bodily functions until recovery.

Oophoritis

Oophoritis is the inflammation of the ovaries, affecting approximately 1 in 15 females who contract mumps after puberty. Symptoms include lower abdominal pain, fever, and nausea. While the condition is usually self-limiting, it can cause significant discomfort during the active phase of the infection.

Mastitis

Mastitis, or inflammation of the breast tissue, can occur in females as a complication of mumps. It may cause breast pain, swelling, and tenderness. Similar to other mumps-related complications, mastitis is typically a temporary condition that improves with the resolution of the underlying mumps infection.

Encephalitis and Meningitis
Encephalitis, inflammation of the brain, and meningitis, inflammation of the membranes surrounding the brain and spinal cord, are rare but serious complications of mumps. Symptoms can include fever, headache, neck stiffness, and sensitivity to light. These conditions require immediate medical attention, as they can lead to severe neurological damage or even be life-threatening.

Long-Term Effects Like Hearing Loss

Hearing loss is a rare but recognized long-term effect of mumps, occurring in less than 1% of cases. It typically presents as unilateral sensorineural hearing loss, where damage occurs to the sensory cells and nerves responsible for hearing. In most instances, hearing loss is temporary, but it can be permanent in some cases.

Each of these complications underscores the importance of preventive measures, such as vaccination, to protect against mumps and its potential long-term effects. While mumps is now less common due to widespread immunization, understanding these complications remains crucial for healthcare providers and individuals alike.

VI

Prevention Of Mumps

Mumps Vaccination

The shield against mumps is the MMR vaccine, a triumph of modern medicine that confers immunity against measles, mumps, and rubella. This vaccine is a beacon of hope, a protector of childhoods, and a guardian against the complications that mumps can bring. It is usually administered in two doses during childhood, the first between 12 to

15 months of age, and the second between 4 to 6 years of age.

Characteristics

The measles virus vaccination known as MMR is a lyophilized preparation of live, attenuated virus that is derived from Enders' attenuated Edmonston strain and is grown in chick embryo cell culture; mumps virus vaccine live, the Jeryl Lynn strain of mumps virus propagated in chick embryo cell culture; and rubella virus vaccine live, the Wistar RA 27/3 strain of live attenuated rubella virus propagated in WI-38 human diploid lung fibroblasts. Similar to the MMR vaccine, the MMRV vaccine contains the same titer of the measles, mumps, and rubella viruses. In comparison to the single-antigen varicella vaccination, the MMRV vaccine has a higher Oka varicella zoster virus titer, at least 9,772 plaque-forming units (PFU) compared to 1,350 PFU.

The vaccinations, which are available in powder form and require re-constituting using sterile, preservative-free water, are MMR and MMRV. Gelatin can be found in both vaccinations. It is possible to deliver MMR and MMRV vaccines subcutaneously.

Neomycin is a substance included in each dose of the MMR and MMRV vaccine. It contains no adjuvant or preservative.

Vaccination Schedule And Use

The immunization recommendations for the prevention of measles, mumps, and rubella can be implemented with the use of the MMR vaccine or MMRV vaccine. The MMR vaccine is authorized for use in patients who are 12 months of age or older. The MMRV vaccination is licensed for use in individuals 12 months of age and older; those 13 years of age or older should not receive the MMRV vaccine. For children 12 months of age and older, two doses of the MMR vaccine spaced at least four weeks apart are generally advised.

The first dose of the MMR vaccine ought to be given to a child between the ages of 12 and 15 months. Based on earlier findings that certain individuals may not develop an immune response to measles after receiving dose 1, a second dose of the MMR vaccine is advised.

Before a child starts kindergarten or first grade, dose 2 is usually administered to them when they are 4 to 6 years old. Before enrolling in school, all children should have had two doses of the MMR vaccine, the first of which should have been given when the child was 12 months old or older. As soon as four weeks have passed since dosage 1, the second dose of the MMR vaccine may be given.

The MMRV vaccination must be given at least three months apart, however it is acceptable to give dose 2 four weeks after dose 1. When a child is between the ages of 12 and 47 months old, they can receive the first dose of the measles, mumps, rubella, and varicella vaccinations either separately or together.

In contrast to children who receive individual vaccinations for MMR and VAR, those who receive the MMRV vaccine have a about twice higher incidence of febrile seizures. When considering delivering MMRV, healthcare providers must talk to parents about the advantages and disadvantages of each immunization choice.

The first dose of the MMR and VAR vaccines in this age range should be given separately, unless the parent or carer indicates a preference for MMRV. MMRV is generally favored over individual injections of its comparable component vaccinations (i.e., MMR vaccine and VAR vaccine) for the second dose of the measles, mumps, rubella, and varicella at any age and for the first dose at 48 months or older.

Vaccination Of Adults

Adults who were born after 1957 ought to have had at least one dose of the MMR vaccine, unless they have proof of prior immunization with at least 1 dose of measles, mumps, and rubella-containing vaccine or other acceptable presumptive evidence of immunity to these three diseases. Except for health care personnel, For those born before 1957, documented immunity to measles, mumps, and rubella is regarded acceptable.

Because of the high population density, colleges and other post-secondary educational institutions are potential high-risk regions for measles, mumps, and rubella transmission.

Pre-matriculation vaccination requirements for measles immunity have been found to dramatically reduce the risk of measles outbreaks on college campuses where they are introduced and enforced. All students entering colleges, universities, technical and vocational schools, and other institutions for post-high school education should receive two doses of the MMR vaccine or have other acceptable evidence of measles, mumps, and rubella immunity before entry.

Healthcare facilities should implement policies that offer two doses of the MMR vaccine at the appropriate interval for measles and mumps, and one dose for rubella, to unvaccinated healthcare

personnel born before 1957 who do not have laboratory evidence of immunity to the measles, mumps, or rubella, or who do not have laboratory confirmation of the disease. In addition, regulations for such staff members should advise receiving two doses of the MMR vaccine during a measles or mumps outbreak and one dose during a rubella outbreak. This recommendation
is based on serologic studies indicating that among hospital personnel born before 1957, 5% to 10% had no detectable measles, mumps, or rubella antibody. A minimum of one MMR dose for rubella and two correctly spaced MMR doses for the measles and mumps constitute an

adequate vaccination regimen for healthcare workers born in 1957 or later.

Revaccination

A vaccination against the measles, mumps, or rubella virus given before the age of 12 months (for instance, in preparation for a foreign trip) should not be included in the 2-dose series. Children who received their first vaccination before turning 12 months old should receive a second dose of the MMR or MMRV vaccine at least 4 weeks apart. The first dose should be given when the child is between 12 and 15 months old (or 12 months if the child continues to live in an area with a high risk of disease).

Unless they have other viable current options, individuals who suffered prenatal HIV infection and may have received the MMR vaccine before the development of successful combination antiretroviral therapy (cART) should be revaccinated with two suitably spaced doses of MMR (i.e., the dosage does not count). When effective cART has been established for at least six months and there is no sign of significant immunosuppression, the MMR series should be given.

Vaccination During Mumps Outbreaks

It is advised that populations identified by public health authorities as being more susceptible to contracting the mumps receive a third dose of the MMR vaccine during an outbreak in order to enhance immunity against the mumps virus and its associated consequences. Public health officials will let healthcare professionals know which populations are more vulnerable and ought to get a dose of the MMR vaccine. The MMR vaccine should be administered to everyone who is shown to be a member of the group at elevated risk and who is not ineligible for it.

Those without vaccination records attesting to their previous receipt of two doses of the MMR vaccine fall under this category.

Mumps Immunity

In general, a person is immune to the mumps if they were born before 1957, have laboratory confirmation of the illness, have proof of having received a sufficient dose of the vaccine, or have serologic evidence of mumps immunity (ambiguous test findings should be regarded as negative).
Any widely used serologic assay can detect the mumps IgG antibody, which is acceptable proof of immunity to the

mumps but does not guarantee protection from the disease. As a positive IgG titer may suggest acute infection, close contacts of mumps patient(s) should not be screened for laboratory evidence of immunity during an outbreak.

Immunogenicity And Vaccine Efficacy

The mumps vaccine results in a moderate, noncommunicable infection that is inapparent. A single dosage results in detectable mumps antibody development in about 94% of recipients. The single antigen mumps vaccination, MMR vaccine, and MMRV vaccine all have comparable rates of seroconversion. Post Licensure studies determined that vaccine effectiveness of one dose of mumps or MMR vaccine was 78% and two dose mumps vaccine effectiveness is 88%.

- **Avoiding Contact with Infected Individuals**

Mumps is a master of disguise, capable of spreading before symptoms even begin to show. To prevent its stealthy march, one must be vigilant and maintain a respectful distance from those infected. This means abstaining from social events, staying home from work or school, and minimizing contact within the household when possible56.

The act of avoiding contact is a silent solidarity, a collective effort to protect not just oneself but the entire community. It is a practice of mindfulness, where every interaction is weighed for its potential to harm or heal.

- **Regular Hand Washing**

Hand washing, a simple act often taken for granted, is a powerful weapon in the fight against mumps. With soap and water, we can dismantle the virus's attempts to cling to us, to travel with us, to invade others through our touch78. It is a ritual of cleanliness, a barrier that stands firm against the spread of infection.

Regular hand washing is not just about personal hygiene; it's a communal chorus, a shared commitment to health. It's the understanding that our hands, which embrace and build, can also carry unseen threats. By washing them frequently, we ensure that our touch remains a gesture of care, not contagion.

In conclusion, the prevention of mumps is a tapestry of strategies, woven together by vaccines, vigilance, and the very human act of washing hands. It's a narrative of how simple actions, informed choices, and scientific advances can come together to safeguard our health and our futures.

VII

Conclusion

Summary of Key Points

Mumps, an illness that has journeyed through human history, leaving tales of swollen cheeks and school absences in its wake, is a viral disease that primarily affects the salivary glands. It is known for its most striking symptom: the swelling of the parotid glands, which can cause discomfort and a distinctive facial appearance.

The virus spreads through saliva and respiratory droplets, making it highly contagious in close-contact environments. Symptoms typically manifest two to three weeks after exposure and can include fever, headache, muscle aches, fatigue, and the hallmark swollen glands.

Diagnosis is usually based on the presence of these symptoms, particularly the swollen glands, and can be confirmed through laboratory tests such as antibody tests or viral culture3. Treatment, however, is supportive, as the body often clears the virus on its own. Pain relievers, hydration, and rest are the mainstays of symptom management.

The Significance Of Vaccination And Early Treatment

Vaccination stands as the cornerstone of mumps prevention. The MMR vaccine, which also protects against measles and rubella, has led to a dramatic decline in mumps cases worldwide. It is administered in childhood and is highly effective in preventing the disease.

The significance of vaccination cannot be overstated. It not only protects individuals from contracting mumps but also contributes to the broader concept of herd immunity, which safeguards communities and those who cannot be vaccinated due to medical reasons.

Early treatment, while not curative, plays a vital role in mitigating the discomfort caused by mumps and preventing potential complications. Recognizing symptoms promptly and seeking medical advice can ensure that supportive measures are taken early, improving the patient's quality of life during the illness.

In conclusion, mumps is a virus that we have come to understand well through the lens of science and medicine. Its impact on health can be significant, but with the tools of vaccination and supportive care, it is a challenge that humanity can meet with confidence. The story of mumps is one of resilience, a narrative where prevention and care come together to protect the fabric of our health and well-being.

www.ingramcontent.com/pod-product-compliance
Lightning Source LLC
Chambersburg PA
CBHW070411230526
45471CB00006B/2751